T0128573

My Miracle Healing from Type 2 Diabetes in Ninety Days

A True Story

Herbert E. McArthur Sr.

WESTBOW
PRESS®
A DIVISION OF THOMAS NELSON
& ZONDERVAN

WestBow Press books may be ordered through booksellers or by contacting:

WestBow Press
A Division of Thomas Nelson & Zondervan
1663 Liberty Drive
Bloomington, IN 47403
www.westbowpress.com
1 (866) 928-1240

Scripture taken from the New King James Version®. Copyright © 1982 by Thomas Nelson. Used by permission. All rights reserved.

ISBN: 978-1-9736-7976-9 (sc)
ISBN: 978-1-9736-7977-6 (hc)
ISBN: 978-1-9736-7975-2 (e)

Library of Congress Control Number: 2019918278

Print information available on the last page.

WestBow Press rev. date: 12/11/2019

In loving memory of Pastor Edward J. Paine

Contents

Acknowledgments

FIRST AND FOREMOST, I am eternally grateful for my Lord and Savior Jesus Christ: Thank you, Lord, for saving me, and thank you, Lord, for this victory.

Pastor Edward Payne (RIP): He was my spiritual mentor, whom I miss immensely, I will continue to live my life for the Lord, and I know I will see him again someday.

Senior Pastor Bruce Klepp, a very prayerful and godly man, you are our leader, our mentor, and our friend. Thank you, Pastor, for your leadership.

Dolly Cedeno: What a blessing to have you in my life. Your knowledge, expertise, and patience has helped me overcome this disease. Denise and I love you so much. Thank you from the bottom of our hearts.

Kevin Gonzalez: Thank you for working with me each week. You helped me win this battle. I will always be grateful. You are a true professional.

Dr. Antonio Pena: Throughout the years I have been under your medical care; you and your office staff have been like family to me. You have my trust and confidence. Thank you so much.

To my wife, Denise: I absolutely could not have done the work God required of me without your unconditional love and support.

You are my foundation, my strength, and my heart will forever belong to you. I love you.

To my daughter, Rachelle: Thank you for being there for me throughout this journey. You exercised alongside me in our home gym each week. You helped me to stay focused and embraced listening to Christian music while exercising. I love you, baby.

Preface

ACCORDING TO AN article I found on Healthline.com, type 2 diabetes is on the rise internationally. More than four hundred million people are living with diabetes as of 2015. The World Health Organization (WHO) predicts that 90 percent of the people all over the world who have diabetes have type 2. It is estimated that 1.5 million deaths occurred in 2012 from diabetes. Over eight out of ten of these deaths occurred in low- and middle-income countries; in developing nations, a little more than half of diabetes cases go undiagnosed. This article furthermore notes the World Health Organization predicts that deaths related to diabetes will double by the year 2030.[1]

Diabetes is a devastating disease that could cause vision damage, heart attack, stroke and kidney complications as well as nerve damage and Alzheimer's disease. My victory over this disease compelled me to write the details of my journey. I wanted to share how this disease snuck up on me when I least expected it, without any clear warning signs. I wanted to share how determination to get control of my body superseded my daily

---

[1] (https://www.healthline.com/health/type-2-diabetes/statistics#1, second paragraph under Worldwide)

struggle of negative thoughts. To have victory is to overcome something. To fight and overcome, one has to know how to do it, which steps to take, what works, and what does not work. Experience in handling the challenges in our lives is of great value, but I had no such experience in this fight. Each day I prayed for wisdom, researched and sought to educate myself on ways to beat this disease. My prayer for this book is that as you read my story you will be inspired by the process and method I used to battle diabetes.

I'm not saying that this is the answer for everyone. I am simply sharing what God has done for me in an effort to give hope to those who are fighting diabetes. This is my true story as documented in my medical record, including my ninety-day follow-up visit results. The results moved my doctor and led me to praise and glorify the Lord. I can't thank him enough for what he has done for me.

Introduction

ONE OF LIFE'S most humbling experiences are illnesses that we or our family members and friends encounter. I know this first hand because I lost all three of my siblings to sickness and disease. My elder brother suffered a massive stroke at the age of forty-eight years old. He lived for seven years in an almost-vegetative state before he passed away at the age of 55 January 24th 2004. Shortly after he suffered a stroke, I gave my life to Christ. I felt that if I was saved, God would listen to my prayers and save my brother's life; we had a very close relationship, he was my best friend. My youngest sister suffered from kidney failure and after being on dialysis for a while, was called home February of 2011 at the age of 53, 19 days before her 54th birthday. My eldest sister battled cancer for several years and passed away one year after my youngest sister in February of 2012, she was 61 years old. My father passed away due to diabetes-related heart failure in his early fifties. While it is painful to lose loved ones, the pain is even greater when the loss is sudden and unexpected. My mom is still living at the ripe old age of 95 and is doing quite well, thank God.

As a young boy about eleven years old, I attended church and played the piano and sang before the Lord. I didn't know much about the Lord at that age, but I knew I enjoyed singing and playing the piano in church. My parents were members of Mt. Calvary Baptist Church and instilled religious values in me and my siblings' lives. Throughout my adult years, I became a greater believer and slowly learned how to pray. I always believed in God but rarely read his word as I should have, knowing what I know now. After I was saved, I began to study God's word and receive his messages for my life in church. I started to realize how much God loves us and that it is not his will for us to be sick. Isaiah 53:5 tells us "that by his stripes we are healed."

I also began to understand that when we pray and ask God for a miracle, according to James 1:6 "you must believe and not doubt" (NKJV). James 2:26 tells us that "faith without works is dead" (NKJV). Scriptures teach us God's plan and his will for our lives so we can be blessed and be well (Proverbs 4:20–22 NKJV). I believe that reading God's word over the years help to prepare me for that August 2018 diagnosis. As you read further, you will learn more about the diagnosis I received.

If you have ever been on the receiving end of a bad diagnosis, you may know the gut wrenching feeling that comes along with that moment. I can honestly say I did not know the faith, strength, and courage I had within me until this battle. I certainly did not know how difficult it would be both mentally and physically. I want my readers to know my struggle and to know this was not easy to hear and certainly not easy to overcome. But with God almighty, anything is possible if you believe. I believe that God prepared me for this day throughout my life for his Glory. I am a product of God's mercy and unconditional love. I am one of God's many miracles. To God be the glory forever and ever. Amen.

1

My Journey

ON AUGUST 31, 2018, I was diagnosed with type 2 diabetes, a Hemoglobin A1c (HbA1c) of 8.8 percent, and a blood sugar level of 246 mg/dl, all detected from a routine yearly physical. You see, a normal blood sugar level is below 100 mg/dl, and a normal A1c is below 5.7 percent. I had no idea and no symptoms—at least none I recognized. I made frequent visits to the restroom, but I chalked it up to drinking a lot of water. My vision was a slightly blurred, but I thought my glasses needed cleaning. I found out a little later, according to my doctor, these were symptoms of high blood sugar. My triglycerides were high, my kidney function dropped, my vitamin D was very low, and my cholesterol was not normal.

Needless to say, hearing these results left me distraught and speechless. My doctor explained to me I had to begin taking a diabetic medication, a cholesterol pill, and vitamin D. Naturally I was stunned, afraid, and confused, my initial reaction was to refuse to accept the prescriptions from my doctor. I was in denial and refused to accept the fact that I needed the medications. My refusal to accept the medications resulted in a verbal scolding from my doctor. My doctor said "this is a very serious matter" you must take these medications and come back to see him in three months (ninety days). At that time, he would do follow-up blood test to see if the medications he'd prescribed worked properly to lower my blood sugar. He also instructed me to purchase a blood-sugar meter. I reluctantly took the prescriptions and left the doctor's office.

My life was over as far as I was concerned. How could this have happened to me? I went to the pharmacy later that day to fill the prescriptions and pick up the blood-sugar meter. The pharmacist said they would not have the medications ready until the next day and would call me when it was ready for pick up. I picked up the blood-sugar meter and went home.

My mind was racing at one hundred miles per hour. Where did I go wrong? Did I eat too much of the wrong things? That night I researched each medication prescribed and found that some diabetic medications were linked to causing pancreatic cancer. I declared to myself "I do not want any type of cancer in my body, therefore I'm going to have to get this done my own." I googled, "Can type 2 diabetes be reversed?" One of my searches indicated it was possible to have it reversed, in fact, it stated it could be reversed with an extreme effort. Although it did not offer details of what the "extreme effort" entailed, but I automatically assumed it entailed a drastic change in eating habits.

I knew I had to return to my doctor's office for a follow-up visit within three months (ninety days). Since I refused to take the diabetic medication, I knew I had to do whatever it took to get better and I had three months to get it done. I realized I had an enormous task ahead and I had to give it my all. I knew deep down inside that one of the reasons my blood sugar was out of control, was because of my eating habits, so the very next day I made an appointment with a registered dietician/nutritionist, Dolly Cedeno.

Dolly treated me a few years before for a condition unrelated to blood sugar, so I trusted her judgment. I met with Dolly a few days later, she began to explain that my diabetes was directly related to what, when, and how I was eating; my lack of exercise and sleep; my weight gain; and my level of stress. She performed a body composition test, weighed me, and then sat me down to ask questions about the types of foods I was eating for breakfast, lunch, and dinner. I responded with the foods I typically ate, including what I ate for snacks or between my meals. After I shared my bad eating habits, she asked me with raised eyebrows, "What time do you normally eat dinner?"

Well, I told her that most of the times I ate around nine o'clock at night. Then she asked me how much sleep I typically get per night. I responded by telling her I went to bed most nights around midnight and would wake up frequently to use the restroom. It appeared as though I was only getting about six hours of sleep per night. We then discussed stress and whether or not I had a lot of stress in my life, and if so, why? After I answered all of her questions and watched her write my responses down, I realized she would use this information to game plan to help me fight this battle. Proper nutrition, exercise, proper sleep, and stress reduction was this recipe for success? I affectionally called these the "big four" and began to research each of them, that evening when I returned home. The next chapter includes some of what I found.

2

My Research and findings on the "Big Four"

(Proper Nutrition)

A GOOD DIET can help minimize the danger of some diseases and health problems: coronary heart disease, diabetes, stroke, some cancers, osteoporosis, high blood pressure, and high cholesterol are just a few. It also enhances your well-being and your capability to combat illnesses.[2] We have all heard about eating healthy and how proper nutrition is the key to good health; this is not a secret. We are told over and over again to eat plenty of vegetables, a portion of fruits, more fish, and some chicken; we are likewise told to drink plenty of water and stay away from too much sugar, right?

---

[2] tuftsmedicarepreferred.org https://www.tuftsmedicarepreferred.org/healthy-living/managing-your-care/diabetes-disease-you-can-manage

Why don't most people adhere to eating properly? It's a mystery. If all nutritional articles and books tell us that we can prevent or cure diseases by eating properly, then why are so many people diagnosed with so many diseases every single day? As you read further, you will notice that I was one of those individuals who knew the benefits of good nutrition but somewhat ignored it. Especially since this disease had already shown its ugly head hereditarily with my dad. I should have paid more attention to my diet and fitness. Because I did not, I paid the price and almost became a statistic of what is often referred to as a preventable disease. According to the World Health Organization, "Over a million died from diabetes alone in 2012."[3] I am convinced that if half of that population would have changed their diet, they would have prevented their own demise.

Dolly says it doesn't cease to amaze her "how food politics are involved in our food choices; food producers care more about their profits rather than our health. There are over three hundred food additives that have been approved by the government and are considered safe" (Dolly Cedeno). We are the only industrialized nation that adds so many chemicals to our food. The word *natural* on a food label doesn't mean "healthy" (Cedeno). Changes to the food label must be approved by Congress. The only way to know if you are eating healthy is by nutrition education. Fortunately, some insurance companies are covering nutrition education as preventative care.

The future doesn't look promising for Americans' health. Statistics suggest that parents are outliving their children due to encouraging an unhealthy lifestyle in their kids. Dolly told me, "Approximately 85 percent of the adult population is considered either overweight or obese" (Cedeno). Four of the ten leading causes of death are related to diet. One third of premature deaths

---

[3] Martino, World Health Organization (2016).). (https://www.healthline. com/health/type-2-diabetes/statistics#1) Article.

in the United States are attributable to poor nutrition and physical inactivity. Americans are consuming diets high in saturated fats, trans fats, salt, and refined sugars. In the last four decades, daily caloric intake has increased by approximately five hundred calories on average. To quote Dolly again, "10 percent of the American population eat a healthy diet. That is approximately 35 million people out of 350 million people in the United States (Cedeno).

It is surprising to most individuals that normal body weight does not guarantee a healthy body. When a person decides to embark on a healthy lifestyle, that individual must keep in mind that muscle mass is the determinant factor of good health. According to Dolly, "Weight does not necessarily correlate with good health. An individual can have a body mass index of thirty; this means that an individual is obese. If the individual body composition is 80 percent muscle mass and 20 percent body fat, that individual is not obese" (Cedeno). Keep in mind that the more muscle mass, the higher the metabolism and the more fat burned.

Dolly explained, too much body fat can be damaging: "High body fat has been associated with obesity, which is associated with an array of disease conditions, such as heart disease, cancers, diabetes, metabolic syndrome, hormone imbalance, and other chronic diseases. Taking care of your body entails eating foods that are free of genetically modified organisms [and] chemicals such as glyphosate (a chemical found in our food supply that can cause cancer)" (Cedeno). "A healthy diet includes vegetables, fruits, whole grains, protein, and healthy fats" (Cedeno). Unfortunately, by the time an individual consults with a nutritionist or a dietitian, it is usually to help manage a disease or condition instead of meeting to discuss prevention strategies. Dolly tells her patients, "If the food was not available one hundred years ago, try not to eat it. The possibility of that food getting you sick is high" (Cedeno). Yes, eating healthy might be expensive, but treatment for a disease or condition is much costlier. It's all about eating foods high in nutrients.

Dolly also states, "If a food product has more than five ingredients, then the product has too many added chemicals. In the 1980s, dietitians recommended margarine instead of butter. Food scientists convinced healthcare providers that margarine was healthier fat than real butter. We learned that margarine increases cholesterol and also causes inflammation to the body" (Cedeno). She further explained, "Healthy nutrition includes high-quality healthy foods (veggies, fruits, and whole grains) that increase energy and reduce inflammation. Inflammation is the main culprit in disease conditions like high blood sugar" (Cedeno).

According to Dolly, the foods that are the most inflammatory to the body are high-fructose corn syrup and partially hydrogenated oils. High-fructose corn syrup acts like alcohol to the body without the buzz (Cedeno). She has treated patients with debilitating conditions as a result of inflammation in the body. After two weeks on a healthy meal plan and a few supplements to support their gut health, their pain and inflammation are significantly reduced. Her advice is, "In your quest to maintain health or to manage a disease condition, it is important to know that healthy eating is a lifetime commitment." The idea is to eat high-quality healthy foods that increase energy, reduces inflammation, and restores health and vitality. Dolly says, "Persistence, perseverance, and determination play an important role in your success to a healthy life" (Cedeno).

3

Exercise

THE DEPARTMENT OF Health and Human Services recommends these exercise guidelines: get at least one hundred and fifty minutes of moderate aerobic activity or seventy-five minutes of vigorous aerobic activity per week, or achieve a mixture of moderate and vigorous activity.[4]

Experts seem to agree that exercise plays a vital role in fighting health conditions and diseases. They state that regular exercise helps combat a wide range of health problems and diseases, such as type 2 diabetes, high blood pressure, stroke, and depression. Being active also keeps the blood flowing smoothly, which decreases the chance of cardiovascular diseases.

I gained a better understanding of what vigorous and moderate exercise meant as I continued to do my research. I sought to understand the physical demands of what would be required of me. To name a few, vigorous activity examples include but

---

[4] mayoclinic.org. https://www.mayoclinic.org/healthy-lifestyle/fitness/expert-answers/exercise/faq-20057916

are not limited to: running, aerobic dance and circuit resistance weight training. While walking, biking, and swimming would be considered more moderate, according to the Harvard School of Public Health.[5] I have engaged in various vigorous and moderate exercises over the years, but not consistently; I've taken days and even weeks off at a time. A body in motion stays in motion; you know the saying. Although sitting and resting are necessary, it is not healthy to habitually sit. The body needs movement and activity to stay strong and healthy.

Kevin Gonzalez, a personal trainer, whom I will formally introduce to my readers later in the book, say's "The average adult person should participate in three to five, one-hour workouts per week. Adults should focus on strengthening workouts at least two to three times a week and cardio or anaerobic training at least two and a half hours per week, specifically in twenty-to-thirty-minute cardio sessions, in order to increase cardiovascular health (Kevin Gonzalez). He also explained that the most important types of resistance exercises are compound movements (bench press, dumbbell curls, etc.), because they use multiple muscles in each repetition and can, therefore, create more resistance. For beginners, it is important to work at a high repetition range until the form is correct in order to prevent injury.

---

[5] hsph.harvard.edu. https://www.hsph.harvard.edu/obesity-prevention-source/moderate-and-vigorous-physical-activity/

4

Sleeping

EVEN ONE NIGHT of missed sleep can create a prediabetic state in an otherwise healthy person.[6]

Getting enough sleep has many benefits. It can help you: get sick less often, stay at a healthy weight, lower your risk for serious health problems, like diabetes and heart disease.[7]

According to Dolly, "Another factor that increases inflammation is the lack of sleep. Sleep is important in promoting health. We have a biological clock that regulates sleep and awake cycles. This cycle helps us regenerate our bodies. When we are chronically sleep-deprived, many of our metabolic processes get disrupted, and this can lead to many chronic diseases, such as diabetes, obesity, depression, cardiovascular disease, Parkinson's

---

[6] hopkinsmedicine.org https://www.hopkinsmedicine.org/health/wellness-and-prevention/the-science-of-sleep-understanding-what-happens-when-you-sleep

[7] "Get Enough Sleep," *Everyday Healthy Eating* (July 18, 2019): https://healthfinder.gov/HealthTopics/Category/everyday-healthy-living/mental-health-and-relationship/get-enough-sleep.

disease, Alzheimer's disease, autoimmune diseases. The number of hours of sleep recommended goes according to age; generally it is between seven and nine hours. It is imperative that your sleep environment is conducive to sleeping."

5

Stress

MENTAL OR EMOTIONAL stress has a combination of effects, depending on the type of diabetes you have. Type 1 diabetes: Mental stress can elevate or decrease blood sugar levels. Type 2 diabetes: Mental stress often elevate blood sugar levels.[8]

At the time I was experiencing a significant amount of pressure over a period of about seven months prior to my diagnosis. Most of this stress derived from my work environment. I worked in a very challenging environment and was under duress almost daily. I knew I had to get out of that situation, so I prepared to retire and did. In addition, I was stressed at home as a result of having to take care of an elderly relative. Our loved ones are important to us, and we want the best for them; no one can take care of them like family. Even though caring for elderly relatives is the right thing to do, it can become an overly stressful situation to be in. It is said, that smiling twenty times a day helps reduce stress. So, smile and be happy.

---

[8] "How Stress Affects Blood Sugar Levels" (2019): https://glucerna.com/why-glucerna/how-stress-affects-blood-sugar-levels.

6

My Journey
Continued: Time
for a Change

I CAN HONESTLY say that all four of these areas in my life needed improvement. I knew all of it had to change, and change pretty quickly. Dolly began to show me my body composition results and discuss how much I weighed. The composition report showed my body fat content verses that of my muscle makeup and other factors. That report substantiated my bad eating habits and nutrition. She illustrated to me on a chart to explain how excess body fat supports diseases and how decreasing fat and adding more muscle would be healthier for a person's body. Based on all the information we talked about that day, she put me on a daily personalized meal plan for all my metabolic issues (diabetes, triglycerides, cholesterol, kidneys, and vitamin D deficiency). My visit with her that day was about two and a half hours. She explained that what I was about to do was going to be a lifestyle change, and I would need to follow the meal plan to the letter. I was filled with anxiety and hope at the same time.

I wanted to start the plan right away. So on my way home from her office I purchased all the food listed on the diet plan. I had a long shopping list and was eager to start eating right. It was a complete overhaul from what I had been eating. I was eating cookies, ice cream, cake, candy, fries, rice, potatoes, bread, pasta, drinking soda, and on occasion drinking very sweet and fruity mixed acholic drinks. In the past, I'd felt that the more sugar I could eat or drink, the better. I had been eating poorly for so long, I guess I just had gotten used to it. But guess what? All of that had to change quickly. This was one of the biggest challenges I had ever faced in my life. Even though I knew I had to make great changes, I knew it was going to take more than just a meal plan, and I knew I would need help, but I wasn't sure how to begin. Denise, said to me, "Remember back in 2015 when you had a health issue? What did you do?"

"What did I do?" I asked her.

"Husband, back then, you put together forty three healing scriptures from the Bible and documented prayers for healing that a very well-known evangelist-pastor had tweeted each day as he was battling cancer. Remember," she said, "you read them daily for almost ten months, and the Lord delivered you from that health scare. Go back to them and start reading them again every day until you receive your miracle."

I realized that this was surely where I needed to start, to read God's word about healing. A great peace came over me, and I was ready to battle this disease. I began to read all of my healing prayers and scriptures nightly. Praying those prayers and scriptures daily emboldened me and gave me courage. I felt that I could trust in God's words: "by his son's stripes my body is healed" (Isaiah 53:5 NKJV).

I also reached out to my church for prayer. One of my pastors, Ed Paine, had moved to Alaska but would come back to Miami every so often. I told my wife instead of going up to the altar I wanted to wait until he returned and let him pray for me. He was my pastor, mentor, and good friend. I had known him for over twenty-three years. Over the years he prayed for many situations in my life, he officiated our wedding, he attended all of my siblings' funerals, and he came to bless every single home I had ever moved into. I felt we had a special connection and that God listened to him when he prayed. He was a special person and loved by all, so I waited until he returned. One Sunday, after he preached, I went to the altar, where he prayed for me. He returned to Alaska and a few months later, we got the news that God had called him home, and our hearts were broken. This was a devastating loss for me, our family, the church family and the community, but I knew he would have wanted me to stay in my faith and keep fighting. May he rest in peace.

I began to reach out to the Lord with prayer and supplication, and God provided me with his master plan for my healing. I started listening to what God was putting in my heart and what it was going to take to get this victory. I had the prayers and scriptures, I received prayer at the altar with Pastor Ed, and I had my meal plan. Now I needed to put together a workout routine. I began to do some cardio on my treadmill and strengthening exercises with my hand weights. It was okay, but I felt like I was not getting the most out of my workout routine and I needed professional help. So after about four weeks of exercising on my own, I hired Kevin Gonzalez, a personal trainer who worked out of Rampant Personal Training and Fitness Studio Body Code in Miami, Florida.

Kevin composed an eight-week training program designed to target all muscle groups, mixed with cardio, six days a week. This was a challenging workout program! I was hoping it would accomplish everything it was designed to do. This was a custom-designed workout routine for my needs and is not intended for everyone.

I started to ensure I was getting at least seven or eight hours of sleep per day and, to the best of my ability, reduce stress in my life. Now that I had the prayers/scriptures, the meal plan, my pastor's prayer, my professional exercise program, and the knowledge to try to get more sleep and reduce my stress levels, I felt I was ready to embark on this journey of eliminating diabetes from my body. Next, I wanted to find out more about trying to lower my blood sugar, if possible, naturally. So my research began.

7

Lowering Blood
Sugar Naturally

I BEGAN TO research how to lower blood sugar naturally. Working with Dolly via text messages and googling information online, I found that there are foods, herbs, and spices that claim to help lower blood sugar naturally. For example, I discovered a spinach and kale smoothie drink that provides more fiber. Fiber helps control blood sugar by slowing down absorption, which helps improve blood sugar levels. Herbs like dill weed, garlic, black pepper, cinnamon, parsley, turmeric, and ginger also help regulate blood sugar. Some beverages, such as chamomile tea, green tea, and apple cider vinegar mixed with water, also lower blood sugar naturally. In my desperation I was trying to get every advantage and all the knowledge I could to help me in this fight to reverse this terrible disease. I discussed all of my findings with Dolly, who encouraged me to begin taking the herbs and drinking teas I found. But my research brought me an even greater discovery, a discovery that is not well known and seldom used to combat diabetes. A Chinese melon that fights high blood sugar naturally and is called "bitter melon". That's right! It's really called bitter melon. It is the most bitter tasting fruit I have ever tasted in my life, but it was the catalyst in bringing my blood sugar under control.

How Does Bitter Melon Affect Diabetes?

According to diabetes.co.uk, "This melon contains at least three active substances with anti-diabetic properties, including charantin, which has been affirmed to have a blood glucose-lowering effect, vicine and an insulin-like compound referred to as polypeptide-p. These substances either work individually or together to help blood sugar levels."[9] Please read the entire article at your leisure (see footnote). Due to copyright constraints I can only share a portion of the article but I guarantee it will be worth reading.

After reading the sentence: "These substances work together or individually to help reduce blood sugar." I was filled with immense hope and excitement that I could barely contain my thoughts. Was this the answer I'd been searching for? Would it work for me? I was truly anxious to try this wonderful fruit. I immediately sought information on how to consume it. It turns out bitter melon has been used for years in the Chinese and Indian cultures to control and regulate blood sugar. Each day I would choose four bitter melons, (which resembles a cucumber). I washed them, slice them horizontally down the middle and remove the seeds. Afterwards, I would feed each slice through the juicer. I'd place the juice in the refrigerator to cool off and let the froth settle for approximately two hours or more. Four bitter

---

[9] "Bitter Melon and Diabetes," Diabetes.co.uk: The Global Diabetes Community: https://www.diabetes.co.uk/natural-therapies/bitter-melon.html.

melons typically produced fourteen to sixteen ounces of juice. Once it cooled down and the froth was removed I would take a sip, about every two hours throughout the day up until bedtime. While it was an extremely unpleasant bitter taste, I figured I would eventually get use to the taste. Boy was I wrong! I still struggle with its bitterness but the benefits certainly outweigh my dislike of the taste. I am a firm believer that juicing bitter melon played a major role in my quest to beat this disease, and Dolly concurs. I juiced this melon and drank it every day for ninety days, and I still juice it today. Please refer to chapter 10 for additional information about lowering blood sugar naturally.

It is important to understand that while proper nutrition and getting yearly physical exams are critical to maintaining good health, you also must include the word of God as a part of your day every day. We are reminded of this in *(Proverbs 4:20–22 NKJV)*: *"My son, attend to my words; consent and submit to my sayings. Let them not depart from your sight; keep them in the center of your heart. For they are life to those who find them, healing and health to all their flesh"*. God is asking us to read and obey his word. He wants us to memorize and keep his words etched in our hearts. In this way, his word promises to give life and health to our bodies. It's just that simple.

In chapter (8) I will share with you my daily prayers and scriptures that reinforced my faith, courage and strength to overcome this disease. I will share the basics of my personal meal plan that worked to reboot and restore me from the inside out. I will disclose how I combined herbs, supplements, juicing, teas, healthy fats, fiber to overcome this disease in ninety days. Lastly, I will describe how my daily exercise routine transformed my physique from a high tendency to store fat to a muscular fat burning machine, which derived from an 8-week personal training program. I want each person to understand that this was a radical and consistent daily effort that took discipline; it was inspired by faith and the belief that "I can do all things through Christ who strengthens me" (Philippians 4:13). Each day represented a new battle and struggle. The hardest part was having to make drastic changes to every part of my life and be consistent. For the most part I was mentally exhausted from trying to get it right and trying to do a combination of things to the best of my ability, because regardless of whether I failed or succeeded I wanted to do my best. I went through so many highs and lows. Each time I measure my blood sugar levels, it would fluctuate up and down. My blood sugar was rarely consistent, this drove me crazy for lack of understanding why. As a result, I drove my wife Denise crazy, until she finally challenged me to simply relax and encouraged me to continue praying, working hard and stop stressing over daily blood sugar levels. She said slow and steady will win the race. I took her message to heart and continued to pray, eat well and exercise. Until this day, I thank her for her unwavering support and sensible encouraging words.

Knowing how important my eating habits would be to my overall success of lowering my blood sugar, I was always on edge about whether or not I was making the right choices when it came to eating out or away from home. I found myself texting Dolly on occasion day and night for advice . I began asking her basic questions such as "can I eat a certain food at a restaurant? "Can I eat anything after 7:00 p.m.?" I would text her daily with what I had eaten the day before. I reported what my blood sugar reading was at bedtime and first thing the following morning. Today, I am beyond grateful for Dolly's patience with me and being there for me throughout one of the most difficult times in my life. She a true friend, and she is like family to me.

As I mentioned in the beginning of the book I did not take any of the prescribed high blood sugar medication, including a pill prescribed to help me normalize my cholesterol. I refused to take them simply because of one of them was linked to pancreatic cancer. This was the deciding factor for me to find an alternative natural way to lower my blood sugar. Throughout this journey,

God revealed time and time again, that prayer is powerful and that faith *with works* is not dead. I am eternally grateful for his grace and mercy. My prayer is that you are blessed by my story and encouraged to believe in God for your miracle healing, for he is able to heal and perform miracles. To God be the glory!

8

Healing Prayers

BEFORE INTRODUCING THE prayers and scriptures below, I'd like to share my heartfelt thoughts on prayer. While all of the other actions I took to fight this disease were absolutely necessary and were in line with having "works" to go with faith, I felt that prayer was my way of letting the Lord know that I believed in his ability to make me whole again. I trusted he would protect me and be with me in times of trouble, as it says in Psalm 91:14–15. Since this was a time of trouble for me and I truly needed God's healing, I prayed and read the scriptures outlined below every single day. To me this was the most important thing I did for my healing. In gratefulness, I continue to read these prayers and scriptures to this day. I pray that these prayers and scriptures serve you in your time of need. I pray that the Lord hears your prayers and heals your body, just as he did for me.

Prayed Daily for Ninety Straight Days

The six prayers below are tweets posted to Twitter in 2015 by @RealRodParsley. I share them here with his permission. Each paragraph denotes a new prayer.

Almighty God, I remain under Your shadow. Jehovah-Rapha, the Lord my Healer, is my refuge and fortress. Your Word is my shield. I'm trusting in Your care and protection. Malachi 4:2 says there is healing in Your wings. Therefore, I am not afraid of disease or any other ungodly thing that would try to harm me. I'm abiding under the shadow of Your protective covering. No plague shall come near my dwelling or my body. I refuse to be sick, in the name of the Lord Jesus Christ. Sickness cannot trespass in my body, because my body is the temple of the Holy Spirit. Sickness [name your sickness] you can't come near me! I resist you! In Jesus name.

Lord Jesus Christ, you have redeemed me by Your blood—I have been ransomed from captivity. Your Word declares that I have been delivered from the authority of Satan and am under Your authority. God, I am free from Satan's dominion, therefore I cannot be dominated with sickness and disease. I have passed out of the devil's jurisdiction, and have been transported into Your Kingdom, the Kingdom of God. I am no longer subject to Satan's authority. I refuse to passively accept sickness and disease. My hope is in the Kingdom of Jehovah-Rapha, the Lord who heals me. My inheritance is healing. I am delivered from Satan and his works. I am free from sickness and disease.

Heavenly Father, I thank you for the fact that I have been crucified with the Lord Jesus Christ. By dying with Him, I have become dead to sickness and disease, and so they can no longer affect my body. Lord Jesus Christ, you are the crucified and resurrected Healer, who lives in me. Therefore, healing is in me. Hallelujah!

Lord Jesus Christ, your name is greater than sickness. You conquered sin, sickness, and Satan (demons, depravity, disease), and in Your name, I command disease to leave my body. Satan, take your hands off my body! I cast you out in the name of Jesus! In the name of Jehovah Joshua Messiah, I am free!

Almighty God, thank You for giving me the tongue of the learned and for awakening my ear to listen. According to Mark 11:22–24 I can have what I say, therefore I declare that You are my Healer. You take sickness away from me, and no evil thing can come close to me. You heal all my diseases. I speak health to every tissue and cell in my body. I release the healing power of God into my being with my words. I also praise You for the ability to listen and as I do, like Jesus, I grow in wisdom, in stature, and in favor daily with You and all people. Thank You, Father.

Lord Jesus Christ, surely You have borne my sickness and diseases and carried my pains. You took my sicknesses on Yourself and carried my pains. You bore them and carried them away to a distance. I don't have to bear what You bore for me! I refuse to bear what You bore for me!

Satan cannot put on me what You bore for me. By Your stripes, I am healed. By Your stripes, I got healing. By your bruises, there is healing for me. Your punishment has brought me healing. Healing has been granted to me. With the stripes that wounded You, I am healed and made whole. I am made whole by the blows You received. My diseases went to the Cross with You and died with You there. Satan, you're visiting the wrong one. Jesus took my sicknesses; and by His stripes, I am healed.

Pray these Bible verses as well:

"Jesus knew their thoughts and said to them: 'Any kingdom divided against itself will be ruined, and a house divided against itself will fall'" (Luke 11:17 NKJV).

"Do you not know that your body is the temple (the very sanctuary) of the Holy Spirit Who lives within you, whom you have received [as a Gift] from God? You are not your own" (1 Corinthians 6:19 NKJV).

Herb's Prayer

Based on the above scriptures, here is my own prayer, also prayed daily:

Heavenly Father, in the name of Jesus, thank you for your word in Luke 11:17 and 1 Corinthians 6:19, for I know the Holy Spirit resides in me, Lord; therefore, sickness or disease cannot live in me, according to your word. My body is the temple of the Lord (1 Corinthians 6:19). Greater is he that is in me than he that is in this world.

My body is the Lord's temple, and this temple, my body, being the temple (house) of the Lord, is not divided against itself; therefore, sickness or disease must go and cannot survive in my body, which is the temple of the Lord. In Jesus's name, I pray. Amen and amen.

Thirteen More Prayers

The thirteen prayers below are also original tweets posted to Twitter in 2015 by @RealRodParsley, which I pray daily as well. I share them with his permission. Again, each paragraph denotes a new prayer.

Lord, I know that sickness is a form of the devil's oppression. I have been delivered from the devil's authority through your Word in Colossians 1:13 (NKJV; "He has delivered us from the power of darkness and has transferred us into the kingdom of His dear Son"). So, I rebuke Satan and every sickness and disease. Healing is mine! The same power that raised Jesus from the dead is at work in me. Healing power is at work in me *now*, and I am free!

Heavenly Father, I submit myself to You. I commit myself to do Your will. I accept Your authority and the authority of Your Word. I resist the devil and all of his works. I stand on Your Word. I stand steadfast and immovable against sickness in Your name, Lord Jesus Christ, I refuse to accept sickness. Disease, you must flee from my body now. Amen.

Lord Jesus Christ, you gave me authority over all of the power of the enemy. Sickness is a sign of the power of the devil; it is my enemy, and I have authority over it. Sickness, you have no right to dominate me—so get out of my body in the name of Jesus! Sickness and disease are under my feet because (Ephesians 2:6 NKJV) says that I am NOW seated with Jesus Christ in heavenly places above all the power of the enemy. Thank You, Jesus, for the victory we have through the power of Your blood and Your sacrifice on the cross of Calvary.

Lord God, my body was not created by You to enable me to sin or to be sick. My body was made to serve You, Lord, and it belongs to You. My body is Your temple, Jehovah-Rapha—You are the Lord who heals. You are healing me now. The blood of Jesus Christ, Jehovah Joshua Messiah, has cleansed me from all sin, and by His stripes, my body is healed. I glorify You, God, in my body by refusing to allow disease to remain. You foul disease, you have no right to remain in my body— get out *now* in the name of the Lord Jesus Christ.

Heavenly Father, I believe I have received my healing. You have healed me! Your Word does not contain truth—it is truth. You have healed me with Your Word, and it is an absolute, accomplished fact. I refuse to consider how my body feels. Pain, sickness, disease, torment, affliction: you have no place in my body, my soul or my spirit! Flee from me now—run away in disgrace! I believe I am healed because You have healed me.

Heavenly Father, you have declared, "I am the Lord who heals you." You are watching over this Word to perform it. You are healing me now. Your Word is full of healing power, and I receive that power now. Your Word has the ability to produce what it says. Healing is part of Your nature. You are in me. Because You live inside of me, Your healing power is at work in me. You are my Shepherd, and I do not lack any good thing, including healing. My body is in contact with You, the Lord who heals me, and it must respond to Your healing life and nature that is at work in me. Healing is in You, and You are in me, according to John 17. Thank You, Father, because You are my healer, and You are healing me now. In Jesus name, I pray, Amen.

Heavenly Father, the prayer of faith has made me whole. I cannot stay down, because You are raising me up! I believe I received when I prayed. I prayed the prayer of faith, and my faith makes me whole. I believe I have received my healing! I am healed.

Heavenly Father, you sent Your Word to heal me and deliver me. Your Word frees me from all corruption. Your Word says that it contains Your ability to perform what it says. Your Word is healing me now. Your Word contains Your healing power. Your Word is working in me now, causing healing to be manifested in my body. I rebuke the thief who comes only to steal, kill and destroy. He has no authority here, because the Lord Jesus Christ came to give me abundant life, and I gratefully receive it.

Lord Jesus, there is power in Your name! You are the resurrected healing Lord. Therefore, in Your Name, I command disease to leave my body.

My body *is* healed in the name of Jesus! I believe according to Acts 3:16 that through faith in His Name, my body is perfectly sound. I am healed in the name of the Lord Jesus Christ.

Bless the Lord, Jehovah Rapha, O my soul. Blessed be God the Father. Lord, I thank You and praise You for Your benefits. You forgive all my sins, all my faults, all my failures, and disobedience. You heal all my diseases, and I thank You for it. Healing belongs to me as part of the New Covenant. Healing is my redemptive right. Thank You, Father, for healing all my diseases.

Precious Lord Jesus Christ, by Your stripes I am healed. Healing belongs to me. I was healed 2,000 years ago by the stripes You bore. It was solely because of Your stripes that I was healed. I'm not trying to get healing; I already have my healing, because Your stripes made my healing possible. I am healed.

Precious Lord Jesus Christ, you have redeemed me from the curse of the Law. You have bought me back, brought me back and set me free from the curse of the Law. Sickness and disease are part of the curse of the Law; therefore, you have redeemed me from all sickness and all disease. I am liberated! I am ransomed! I am free from disease! I am redeemed from every disease written in the curse of the Law, and from every disease that is not written in the Book of the Law. I thank You that You have redeemed me, that I may be free from all sickness and disease. In Jesus name, I pray, Amen.

Heavenly Father, Your Spirit is residing in me at this very moment and is making His home in my spirit. Your Spirit is healing me and is creating life—supplying life in my body and making it whole. The life of Jehovah-Rapha is being applied to my body by Your Spirit dwelling in me. Your life is driving out every trace of sickness and disease in my body. Thank you, Heavenly Father, that Your life is destroying disease and germs in my body right now.

9

Healing Scriptures

I Read These Verses Daily for Ninety Days

1. "If you diligently heed the voice of the Lord your God and do what is right in His sight, give ear to His commandments and keep all His statutes, I will put none of the diseases on you which I have brought on the Egyptians. For I am the Lord who heals you" (Exodus 15:26 NKJV).

2. "Now see that I, even I, am He, and there is no God besides Me; I kill and I make alive; I wound and I heal; Nor is there any who can deliver from My hand" (Deuteronomy 32:39 NKJV).

3. "If My people who are called by My name will humble themselves, and pray and seek My face, and turn from their wicked ways, then I will hear from heaven and will forgive their sin and heal their land" (2 Chronicles 7:14 NKJV).

4. "O Lord my God, I cried out to You, And You healed me" (Psalm 30:2 NKJV).

5. "Have mercy on me, O Lord, for I am weak; O Lord, heal me, for my bones are troubled" (Psalm 6:2 NKJV).

6. "Bless the Lord, O my soul; And all that is within me, bless His holy name! Bless the Lord, O my soul, and forget not all His benefits: Who forgives all your iniquities, who heals all your diseases, Who redeems your life from destruction, who crowns you with lovingkindness and tender mercies" (Psalm 103:1–4 NKJV).

7. "He sent His word and healed them, and delivered them from their destructions" (Psalm 107:20 NKJV).

8. "He heals the brokenhearted and binds up their wounds" (Psalm 147:3 NKJV).

9. "Do not be wise in your own eyes; Fear the Lord and depart from evil. It will be health to your flesh, And strength to your bones" (Proverbs 3:7–8 NKJV).

10. "My son, give attention to my words; Incline your ear to my sayings. Do not let them depart from your eyes; Keep them in the midst of your heart; For they are life to those who find them, And health to all their flesh" (Proverbs 4:20–22 NKJV).

11. "But He was wounded for our transgressions, He was bruised for our iniquities; The chastisement for our peace was upon Him, And by His stripes, we are healed" (Isaiah 53:5 NKJV).

12. "Then your light shall break forth like the morning, your healing shall spring forth speedily, and your righteousness

shall go before you; The glory of the Lord shall be your rear guard" (Isaiah 58:8 NKJV).

13. "The Spirit of the Lord God is upon Me, Because the Lord has anointed Me To preach good tidings to the poor; He has sent Me to heal the brokenhearted, to proclaim liberty to the captives, And the opening of the prison to those who are bound" (Isaiah 61:1 NKJV).

14. "Return, you backsliding children, And I will heal your backslidings. Indeed we do come to You, For You are the Lord our God" (Jeremiah 3:22 NKJV).

15. "Heal me, O Lord, and I shall be healed; Save me, and I shall be saved, For You are my praise" (Jeremiah 17:14 NKJV).

16. "'For I will restore health to you and heal you of your wounds,' says the Lord, 'Because they called you an outcast saying: "This is Zion; No one seeks her"'" (Jeremiah 30:17 NKJV).

17. "Behold, I will bring it health and healing; I will heal them and reveal to them the abundance of peace and truth" (Jeremiah 33:6 NKJV).

18. "Come, and let us return to the Lord; For He has torn, but He will heal us; He has stricken, but He will bind us up" (Hosea 6:1 NKJV).

19. "I will heal their backsliding, I will love them freely, For My anger has turned away from him" (Hosea 14:4 NKJV).

20. "But to you who fear My name, The Sun of Righteousness shall arise with healing in His wings; And you shall go out and grow fat like stall-fed calves" (Malachi 4:2 NKJV).

21. "And Jesus went about all Galilee, teaching in their synagogues, preaching the gospel of the kingdom, and healing all kinds of sickness and all kinds of disease among the people" (Matthew 4:23 NKJV).

22. "Then Jesus said to the centurion, 'Go your way; and as you have believed, so let it be done for you.' And his servant was healed that same hour" (Matthew 8:13 NKJV).

23. "When evening had come, they brought to Him many who were demon-possessed. And He cast out the spirits with a word, and healed all who were sick" (Matthew 8:16 NKJV).

24. "Then Jesus went about all the cities and villages, teaching in their synagogues, preaching the gospel of the kingdom, and healing every sickness and every disease among the people" (Matthew 9:35 NKJV).

25. "And when He had called His twelve disciples to Him, He gave them power over unclean spirits, to cast them out, and to heal all kinds of sickness and all kinds of disease" (Matthew 10:1 NKJV).

26. "Heal the sick, cleanse the lepers, raise the dead, cast out demons. Freely you have received, freely give" (Matthew 10:8 NKJV).

27. "Then one was brought to Him who was demon-possessed, blind and mute; and He healed him so that the blind and mute man both spoke and saw" (Matthew 12:22 NKJV).

28. "And when Jesus went out He saw a great multitude; and He was moved with compassion for them, and healed their sick" (Matthew 14:14 NKJV).

29. "And the whole multitude sought to touch Him, for power went out from Him and healed them all" (Luke 6:19 NKJV).

30. The twelve are sent out: "So they departed and went through the towns, preaching the gospel and healing everywhere" (Luke 9:6 NKJV).

31. The seventy are sent out: "Whatever city you enter, and they receive you, eat such things as are set before you. And heal the sick there, and say to them, 'The kingdom of God has come near to you'" (Luke 10:8–9 NKJV).

32. The story of the ten lepers: "And one of them, when he saw that he was healed, returned, and with a loud voice glorified God" (Luke 17:15 NKJV).

33. "So when Peter saw it, he responded to the people: 'Men of Israel, why do you marvel at this? Or why look so intently at us, as though by our own power or godliness we had made this man walk?'" (Acts 3:12 NKJV).

34. Healing of the lame man at the Gate Beautiful: "Now, Lord, look on their threats, and grant to Your servants that with all boldness they may speak Your word, 'by stretching out Your hand to heal, and that signs and wonders may be done through the name of Your holy Servant Jesus.' And when they had prayed, the place where they were assembled together was shaken; and they were all filled with the Holy Spirit, and they spoke the word of God with boldness" (Acts 4:29–31 NKJV).

35. "To another faith by the same Spirit, to another, gifts of healings by the same Spirit" (1 Corinthians 12:9 NKJV).

36. "Is anyone among you sick? Let him call for the elders of the church, and let them pray over him, anointing him with oil in the name of the Lord. And the prayer of faith will save the sick, and the Lord will raise him up. And if he has committed sins, he will be forgiven. Confess your trespasses to one another, and pray for one another, that you may be healed. The effective, fervent prayer of a righteous man avails much" (James 5:14–16 NKJV).

37. "In the middle of its street, and on either side of the river, was the tree of life, which bore twelve fruits, each tree yielding its fruit every month. The leaves of the tree were for the healing of the nations" (Revelation 22:2 NKJV).

38. "Now when the woman saw that she was not hidden, she came trembling; and falling down before Him, she declared to Him in the presence of all the people the reason she had touched Him and how she was healed immediately" (Luke 8:47 NKJV).

39. "And He said to her, 'Daughter, be of good cheer; your faith has made you well. Go in peace'" (Luke 8:48 NKJV).

40. "Now it happened on a certain day, as He was teaching, that there were Pharisees and teachers of the law sitting by, who had come out of every town of Galilee, Judea, and Jerusalem. And the power of the Lord was present to heal them" (Luke 5:17 NKJV).

41. "The moon will shine like the sun, and the sunlight will be seven times brighter, like the light of seven full days, when the Lord binds up the bruises of his people and heals the wounds he inflicted" (Isaiah 30:26 NKJV).

42.

> But what can I say?
> He has spoken to me, and he himself has done this.
> I will walk humbly all my years
> because of this anguish of my soul.
> Lord, by such things people live;
> and my spirit finds life in them too.
> You restored me to health
> and let me live.
> Surely it was for my benefit
> that I suffered such anguish.
> In your love you kept me
> from the pit of destruction;
> you have put all my sins
> behind your back. (Isaiah 38:15–17 NKJV)

43.

> Whoever dwells in the shelter of the Most High
> will rest in the shadow of the Almighty.
> I will say of the Lord, "He is my refuge and my
> fortress,
> my God, in whom I trust."
> Surely, he will save you
> from the fowler's snare
> and from the deadly pestilence.
> He will cover you with his feathers,
> and under his wings you will find refuge;
> his faithfulness will be your shield and rampart.
> You will not fear the terror of night,
> nor the arrow that flies by day,
> nor the pestilence that stalks in the darkness,
> nor the plague that destroys at midday.

A thousand may fall at your side,
ten thousand at your right hand,
but it will not come near you.
You will only observe with your eyes
and see the punishment of the wicked.
If you say, "The Lord is my refuge,"
and you make the Most High your dwelling,
no harm will overtake you,
no disaster will come near your tent.
For he will command his angels concerning you
to guard you in all your ways;
they will lift you up in their hands so that you will
not strike your foot against a stone.
You will tread on the lion and the cobra;
you will trample the great lion and the serpent.
"Because he loves me," says the Lord, "I will
rescue him;
I will protect him, for he acknowledges my name.
He will call on me, and I will answer him;
I will be with him in trouble,
I will deliver him and honor him.
With long life, I will satisfy him
and show him my salvation." Amen. (Psalm 91
NKJV)

10

My Ninety-Day
Meal Plan

PLEASE NOTE THAT the following meal plan was tailored and customized for me considering my condition based on the recommendations from my nutritionist. This was what worked for me and by no means should be used to remedy your ailment. Again, this was a radical change and consisted of unwavering persistence, determination, hard work, faith, and hope. I pray that this meal plan inspires you to seek expert advice to help you with your nutritional needs.

I strictly followed a daily meal plan that included breakfast, lunch, dinner and snacks. I understood that the purpose of this meal plan was to help eliminate the unhealthy foods I was consuming and begin a healthier diet geared towards the types of foods that would decrease my blood sugar level and regulate it. For example, foods that have a lower glycemic index (GI) are digested slower, causing a smaller rise in blood sugar levels. Refined sugars, such as high-fructose corn syrup and refined grains, usually have a higher GI and are digested and absorbed quicker, resulting in a rapid rise in blood sugar levels.[10] As a result, my nutritionist Dolly, designed a specific meal plan for me to follow daily that included supplements, healthy fats, teas, and herbs. I had to follow this meal plan for 90 days and also for the rest of my life. The first two weeks I consumed nothing but wild-caught fish and vegetables; intended to detox my body. Despite the difficulty of starting a new meal plan, I knew I had to adapt to this new way of eating if I wanted to accomplish my goals.

Here are the staples of my daily plan:

I avoided rice, potatoes, starchy vegetables, high-sugar-content foods, high-carb foods, and snacks at all cost. Highly starchy foods turn into sugars, therefore I avoided them altogether.

Instead I consumed non-starchy vegetables, leafy greens, Ezekiel breads, eggs, healthy fats (such as avocado, seeds, butter, olive oil, nuts, and wild-caught fish) and chicken.

One of My Actual Meals

⬇

Grilled mahi-mahi, steamed broccoli with red onions, cucumber, avocado, olive oil, and apple cider vinegar, sprinkled with dill weed and black pepper.

Other Examples of What I Consumed

Herbs

I consumed these herbs daily: turmeric, ginger, dill weed, renapath, and *bu zhong yi qi tnag*. Both turmeric and ginger help reduce inflammation in the body. Renapath is for kidney support, and bu zhong supports the immune system.

---

[10] healthline.com.

Supplements

I consumed these vitamins as per my nutritionist instructions: vitamin C, vitamin D, vitamin E, omega-3 fatty acids, and magnesium. These are all important supplements for overall body maintenance and care. Vitamin D helped my levels return to normal.

Juicing

Every two hours, seven days a week, I juiced fourteen to sixteen ounces of Chinese bitter melon. Bitter melon contains at least three active substances with anti-diabetic properties and is confirmed to have a blood glucose-lowering effect.

Teas

Each day, I drank green tea, chamomile tea, turmeric tea, and a mixture of apple cider vinegar and water. These beverages are all known to help regulate blood sugar levels.

Healthy Fats

I included one or more of the following healthy fats in every meal: organic butter, avocado, wild-caught fish, seeds, organic olive oil, nuts (a daily snack), nut butter, and olives. A diet rich in the above healthy fats could lower sugar levels.

Fiber

For fiber, I drank a smoothie each morning made of spinach, kale, turmeric, and ginger. Fiber helps control blood sugar by slowing down absorption, which helps improve blood sugar levels. Both turmeric and ginger fight inflammation in the body.

Water

I drank at least six to eight glasses of water daily. Water is vital to the body and it helps regulate sugar.

Lowering Blood Sugar Naturally

I recommend researching how to lower blood sugar naturally, as there is plenty to learn. I highly recommend the work of Franziska Spritzer, RD, CDE.[11] Read all of her Healthline articles. Below I share a small portion of a valuable article. This publication helped me to understand how important it is to learn about how certain foods can help regulate or lower blood sugar naturally and at the same time provide important nutrients for the body.

According to Spritzer's article, here are a few food items that help lower blood sugar:

Salmon, Sardines, Herring, Anchovies
The bottom line is that fatty fish has omega-3 fats that decrease inflammation and other risk factors that may lead to diabetes, heart disease, and stroke.

Leafy Greens
One study showed that increasing vitamin C intake decreased inflammatory markers and fasting blood sugar levels for people with type 2 diabetes.

Cinnamon
Cinnamon intake may improve blood sugar control, insulin sensitivity, cholesterol, and triglyceride levels in type 2 diabetics.

Eggs
Eggs improve risk factors related to heart disease, help promote good blood sugar control, and enhance eye protection.

---

[11] Franziska Spritzer, "The 16 Best Foods to Control Diabetes," Healthline (June 3, 2017): https://www.healthline.com/nutrition/16-best-foods-for-diabetics.

Turmeric

Turmeric contains curcumin, which helps reduce blood sugar levels and inflammation and also protect against heart and kidney disease.

Nuts

Nuts are an excellent, healthy addition to a diabetic diet. They're low in digestible carbs, which helps to reduce blood sugar, insulin, and LDL or Low-density lipoprotein cholesterol levels.

Broccoli

Broccoli is an almost zero-calorie, low-carb, non-starchy food with high nutrients. It can aid in controlling blood sugar.

Extra-Virgin Olive Oil

Extra-virgin olive oil contains healthy oleic acid. Therefore, it is beneficial for blood pressure and a healthier heart. It's one of the good fats that may help in controlling blood sugar.

Flaxseeds

Flaxseeds may decrease inflammation, help lower the risk for developing heart disease, help decrease blood sugar levels, and improve insulin sensitivity.

Apple Cider Vinegar

Apple cider vinegar can improve insulin sensitivity to help lower blood sugar levels.

Garlic

Garlic helps decrease blood sugar, inflammation (a key factor in blood sugar control), LDL cholesterol, and blood pressure in people with diabetes.

Squash

Squash may help decrease blood sugar and insulin levels.

A Few Meal Tidbits

Following this healthy meal plan was a significantly different way of eating for me, and after about two weeks I began to notice a boost in energy and some weight loss. I ate plenty of broccoli and spinach and discovered creative ways to prepare them. Stir-frying these vegetables with organic butter or steaming them with a little olive oil and a touch of Himalayan salt made for a great side dish.

Most of the fish I ate was salmon, but I also ate mahi-mahi, flounder, sardines, and swordfish, all wild-caught. From baked to grilled, it was all delicious.

For a snack, I simply ate nuts and occasionally, strawberries or tangerines.

Avocados became a delight with almost every meal, adding flavor and one of the necessary healthy fats to help fight off the high blood sugar in my body.

The teas similarly helped lower blood sugar naturally.

Supplements, juicing, fats, and fibers also played a factor in lowering blood sugar naturally. I chose not to publish all the specifics of the day-to-day actual meal plans for breakfast, lunch, dinner, and snacks, as it was tailored just for me by my nutritionist. Full recipes of my prepared meals may be available later this year according to demand. In the meantime, I highly recommend consulting with a dietitian who can customize a meal plan for your individual health needs.

11

My Exercise Plan

NOTE: THE FOLLOWING workout plan was explicitly designed for me and my training needs. This workout is not for everyone. Personal training should be personalized by professionals for your individual needs and benefits, as Kevin did for me.

This plan worked amazingly well for me. I was able to achieve being in the best shape of my life and I continue to use this plan to this day. While the workouts were a challenge for me in the beginning, I grew stronger each day and became better at performing the workouts each week. A plan such as this can do the same for you with the support of a professional trainer.

Kevin recommends starting with five to ten repetitions for the first few weeks and slowly working your way to a repetition range between fifteen and twenty-five. Resting for thirty to sixty seconds between sets is also critical, resting helps promote muscle growth. Another challenge introduced later in my training was doing supersets—doing two exercises in a row without rest. This not only promotes muscle growth but also raises the heart rate, especially when done in high repetitions. In the case of resistance workouts, it is important to manage the load so that your muscles are not overworked.

Make sure that each time you train a specific muscle group, the following time you change the repetition range. For example, week 1 perform a chest exercise (bench press) for fifteen reps, week 2 for sixteen reps, and week 3 for twenty reps. Some of the most important exercises during these workouts are body-weight exercises, including push-ups, pull-ups, triceps dips, squats, and lunges. Kevin emphasis the importance of having proper mechanics to perform these exercises, which is why strength plays such an important role early in training. The most important compound exercises during the workouts included barbell bench press, flat dumbbell (DB) press, standing DB press, DB rows, cable rows, bicep curls, squats, and lunges. You may refer to all of the exercises in my eight-week workout plan documented for your review in the next Chapter. Illustrations of each exercise can be found in the appendix.

12

My Eight-Week Workout Plan: Week One

NOTE: ALL OF the listed exercises can be found online, if desired.

Monday: Legs

- Dumbbell squats: 4 × 12 (rest one minute between sets)
- Leg extensions with a two-second hold at the top: 4 × 15 (rest one minute between sets)
- Leg curls with a two-second hold at the top: 4 × 15 (rest one minute between sets)
- Lunges (one leg at a time, holding a dumbbell in each hand): 4 × 15 (switch legs instead of rest)

Tuesday: Upper Body

Same as Friday's upper body workout

Wednesday: Cardio

Cardio of choice: twenty minutes

Thursday: Legs

Same as Monday's leg workout

Friday: Upper Body

Chest
- Flat bench press: 4 × 12 (one-minute rest between sets)
- Pectoral fly with a two-second hold in the middle: 4 × 12 (one-minute rest between sets)
- Eighty push-ups (break into sets and rest as much as you need)

Back
- Thirty pull-ups (break into sets and rest as much as you need)
- Seated row: 4× 12 (one-minute rest between sets)
- One arm dumbbell rows: 4 × 15 (switch arms instead of rest)

Shoulders
- Dumbbell shoulder press: 4 × 12 (one-minute rest between sets)
- Lateral raises: 4 × 15 (one-minute rest between sets)

Triceps
- Triceps push down with bar: 4 × 12 (one-minute rest between sets)
- Triceps dumbbell overhead extensions: 4 × 15 (one-minute rest between sets)

Biceps
- Barbell curls: 4 × 12 (one-minute rest between sets)
- Dumbbell hammer curls two-second hold on top for two seconds: 4 × 15 (one-minute rest between sets)

Saturday: Cardio

Treadmill: twenty minutes

13

Week Two

Monday: Legs

- Dumbbell squats: 5 × 20 (rest forty-five seconds between sets)
- Leg extensions with two-second hold at the top: 5 × 20 (rest forty-five seconds between sets)
- Leg curls with two-second hold at the top: 5 × 20 (rest forty-five seconds between sets)
- Two-legged calf raises

Tuesday: Upper Body

Same as Friday's upper body workout

Wednesday: Cardio

Cardio of choice: twenty-five minutes

Thursday: Legs

Same as Monday's leg workout

Friday: Upper Body

Chest
- Flat bench press: 4 × 15 (rest forty-five seconds between sets)
- Incline dumbbell bench press: 4 × 15 (rest forty-five seconds between sets)
- Chest cable cross: 4 × 15 (rest forty-five seconds between sets)
- Eighty-five push-ups (break into sets and rest as much as you need)

Back
- One-armed dumbbell rows: 5 × 20 (switch arms instead of rest)
- Barbell rows: 5 × 20 (rest forty-five seconds between sets)
- Seated rows: 5 × 20 (rest forty-five seconds between sets)

Shoulders
- Dumbbell shoulder press: 4 × 20 (rest forty-five seconds between sets)
- Lateral raises: 4 × 20 (rest forty-five seconds between sets)
- Frontal raises: 4 × 20 (rest forty-five seconds between sets)

Triceps
- Triceps push down with bar: 4 × 20 (rest forty-five seconds between sets)
- One-armed triceps dumbbell overhead extensions: 4 × 15 (switch arms, no rest)

Biceps
- Barbell curls: 5 × 20 (rest forty-five seconds between sets)
- Dumbbell concentration curls: 5 × 15 (switch hands, no rest)

Saturday: Cardio

- Treadmill: twenty-five minutes

14

Week Three

Monday: Legs

- Static lunges: 4 × 15 (no weight, switching legs for rest)
- Dumbbell squats: 4 × 15 (rest thirty seconds between sets)
- Leg extensions: 4 × 20 (rest thirty seconds between sets)
- Leg curls: 4 × 20 (rest thirty seconds between sets)

Tuesday: Upper Body

Same as Friday's upper body workout

Wednesday: Cardio

Cardio of choice: thirty minutes

Thursday: Legs

Same as Monday's leg workout

Friday: Upper Body

Chest
- Chest cable cross: 4 × 25 (rest thirty seconds between sets)
- Flat dumbbell bench press: 4 × 15 (rest thirty seconds between sets)
- Incline dumbbell bench press: 4 × 15 (rest thirty seconds between sets)
- Ninety push-ups: break into sets and rest as much as you need

Back
- Barbell rows: 4 × 15 (rest thirty seconds between sets)
- Seated rows: 4 × 15 (rest thirty seconds between sets)
- One-armed dumbbell rows: 4 × 15 (rest thirty seconds between sets)

Shoulders
- Lateral raises: 4 × 15 (superset with frontal raises; no rest between sets)
- Frontal raises: 4 × 15
- Seated dumbbell shoulder press: 4 × 15 (forty-five-second rest between sets)

Triceps
- Triceps push down with bar: 4 × 15 (superset with triceps dumbbell overhead extensions; no rest between sets)
- Triceps dumbbell overhead extensions: 4 × 15

Biceps
- Barbell curls: 4 × 15 (rest thirty seconds between sets)
- Hammer curls: 4 × 15 (rest thirty seconds between sets)
- Dumbbell concentration curls: 4 × 15 (switch hands, no rest)

Saturday: Cardio

Treadmill: thirty minutes

15

Week Four

Monday: Legs

- Dumbbell squats: 4 × 20
- Leg extensions with two-second hold: 4 × 15 (rest thirty seconds between sets)
- Leg curls with two-second hold: 4 × 15 (rest thirty seconds between sets)
- Walking lunges: 4 × 15

Tuesday: Upper Body

Same as Friday's upper body workout

Wednesday: Cardio

Cardio of choice: thirty minutes

Thursday: Legs

Same as Monday's leg workout

Friday: Upper Body

Chest
- Flat dumbbell bench press: 4 × 20 (rest thirty seconds between sets)
- Incline dumbbell bench press: 4 × 20 (rest thirty seconds between sets)
- Incline dumbbell fly: 4 × 20 (rest thirty seconds between sets)
- Ninety-five push-ups (break into sets and rest as much as you need)

Back
- Underhand barbell rows: 4 × 20 (rest thirty seconds between sets)
- Seated rows with two-second hold: 4 × 20 (switch arms instead of rest)
- Lateral pulldown: 4x20 (rest thirty seconds between sets)

Shoulders
- Dumbbell shoulder press: 4 × 20 (rest thirty seconds between sets)
- Lateral raises with two-second hold: 4 × 20 (rest thirty seconds between sets)
- Frontal raises with two-second hold: 4 × 20 (rest thirty seconds between sets)

Triceps
- Triceps push down with bar: 4 × 15 (superset with triceps dumbbell overhead extensions; no rest between sets)
- Triceps dumbbell overhead extensions: 4 × 15

Biceps
- Barbell curls: 4 × 15 (superset with hammer curls)
- Hammer curls: 4 × 15 (rest thirty seconds between sets)
- Standing alternating dumbbell curls: 4 × 20 (rest thirty seconds between sets)

Saturday: Cardio

Cardio of choice: thirty minutes

16

Week Five

Monday: Legs

- Leg extensions: 4 × 25 (rest thirty seconds between sets)
- Leg curls: 4 × 25 (rest thirty seconds between sets)
- Dumbbell squats with two-second holds: 4 × 20 (rest thirty seconds between sets)
- Dumbbell stiff leg deadlifts: 4 × 20 (rest thirty seconds between sets)

Tuesday: Upper Body

Same as Friday's upper body workout

Wednesday: Cardio

Stair-climber: thirty minutes

Thursday: Legs

Same as Monday's leg workout

Friday: Upper Body

Chest
- Flat dumbbell bench press: 4 × 25 (rest thirty seconds between sets)
- Flat dumbbell fly: 4 × 25 (rest thirty seconds between sets)
- Incline dumbbell bench press: 4 × 20 (rest thirty seconds between sets)
- One hundred push-ups (break into sets and rest as much as you need)

Back
- Barbell rows: 4 × 15 (superset with seated rows)
- Seated rows: 4 × 15 (rest thirty seconds between super sets)
- Lateral pulldown: 4 × 25 (rest thirty seconds between sets)

Shoulders
- Barbell shoulder press: 4 × 25 (rest thirty seconds between sets)
- Lateral raises: 4 × 15 (rest thirty seconds between sets)
- Frontal raises: 4 × 15 (rest thirty seconds between sets)

Triceps
- Triceps push down with bar: 4 × 25 (rest thirty seconds between sets)
- Triceps dumbbell overhead extensions: 4 × 25 (rest thirty seconds between sets)

Biceps

- Barbell curls: 4 × 25 (rest thirty seconds between sets)
- Hammer curls with two-second hold: 4 × 20 (rest thirty seconds between sets)
- Concentration dumbbell curls: 4 × 20 (no rest; just switch arms)

Saturday: Cardio

Cardio of choice: thirty minutes

17

Week Six

Monday: Legs

- Lunges: 4 × 15 (one leg at a time)
- Dumbbell squats: 4 × 15
- Leg extensions: 4 × 20 (rest thirty seconds between sets)
- Leg curls: 4 × 20 (rest thirty seconds between sets)
- Dumbbell squats with two-second holds: 4 × 20 (rest thirty seconds between sets)

Tuesday: Upper Body

Same as Friday's upper body workout

Wednesday: Cardio

Stair-climber: thirty minutes

Thursday: Legs

Same as Monday's leg workout

Friday: Upper Body

Chest
- Flat dumbbell bench press: 4 × 15 (rest thirty seconds between sets)
- Flat dumbbell fly: 4 × 15 (rest thirty seconds between sets)
- One hundred push-ups (break into sets and rest as much as you need)

Back
- Pull-ups, holding on top for five seconds: 4 × 20
- Barbell rows: 4 × 20
- Seated rows: 4 × 20

Shoulders
- Dumbbell shoulder press: 4 × 25
- Lateral raises: 4 × 20
- Frontal raises: 4 × 20

Triceps
- Triceps push down with bar: 4 × 25 (rest thirty seconds between sets)
- One-armed triceps dumbbell overhead extensions: 4 × 15 (rest thirty seconds between sets)

Biceps
- Barbell curls: 4 × 25 (rest thirty seconds between sets)
- Hammer curls with two-second hold: 4 × 20 (rest thirty seconds between sets)

- Concentration dumbbell curls: 4 × 20 (no rest; just switch arms)

Saturday: Cardio

Cardio of choice: thirty minutes

18

Week Seven

Monday: Legs

- Walking Lunges: 4 × 20 (rest thirty seconds between sets)
- Leg extensions: 4 × 15 (rest thirty seconds between sets)
- Leg curls: 4 × 15 (rest thirty seconds between sets)
- Dumbbell squats with two-second hold: 4 × 12 (rest thirty seconds between sets)

Tuesday: Upper Body

Same as Friday's upper body workout

Wednesday: Cardio

Stair-climber: thirty minutes

Thursday: Legs

Same as Monday's leg workout

Friday: Upper Body

Chest
- One hundred push ups
- Flat dumbbell bench press: 4 × 15 (rest thirty seconds between sets)
- Flat dumbbell fly: 4 × 15 (rest thirty seconds between sets)

Back
- Barbell rows: 4 × 15
- One-armed rows: 4 × 15
- Seated rows: 4 × 15

Shoulders
- Dumbbell shoulder press: 4 × 12
- Lateral raises: 4 × 10
- Frontal raises: 4 × 10

Triceps
- Triceps push down with bar: 4 × 12 (rest thirty seconds between sets)
- One-armed triceps dumbbell overhead extensions: 4 × 12 (rest thirty seconds between sets)
- Dips on bench: 4 × 12

Biceps
- Barbell curls: 4 × 15 (forty-five-second rest)

- Hammer curls (heavy): 4 × 12 (rest thirty seconds between sets)
- Alternating curls: 4 × 20 (rest thirty seconds between sets)

Saturday: Cardio

Cardio of choice: thirty minutes

19

Week Eight

Monday: Legs

- Leg extensions: 4 × 10 (superset with squats)
- Dumbbell squats: 4 × 10 (one-minute rest between sets)
- Leg curls: 4 × 10 (superset with deadlifts)
- Dumbbell stiff-leg deadlifts: 4 × 10 (one-minute rest between sets)
- Static lunges: 4 × 25 (one leg at a time; no rest; just switch legs)

Tuesday: Upper Body

Same as Friday's upper body workout

Wednesday: Cardio

Stair-climber: thirty minutes

Thursday: Legs

- Dumbbell squats: 5 × 8
- Leg curls: 4 × 2 drop sets, 10 reps each
- Leg extension: 4 × 2 drop sets, 10 reps each

Friday: Upper Body

Chest
- Flat dumbbell bench press: 4 × 25 (rest thirty seconds between sets)
- Flat dumbbell fly: 4 × 20 (rest thirty seconds between sets)
- fifty decline push ups

Back
- Barbell rows: 4 × 12
- Seated rows with two-second hold: 4 × 15
- Lateral pulldown: 4x20

Shoulders
- Dumbbell shoulder press: 4 × 20
- Lateral raises: 4 × 20
- Frontal raises: 4 × 20

Triceps
- Triceps push down with bar: 4 × 25 (rest thirty seconds between sets)

- One-armed triceps dumbbell overhead extensions: 4 × 20 (rest thirty seconds between sets)
- Dips on bench: 4 × 15

Biceps
- Barbell curls: 4 × 15 (rest for forty-five seconds between sets)
- Hammer curls (heavy) 4 × 10 (thirty 30 seconds rest)
- Alternating curls 4 × 20 (thirty seconds)

Saturday: Cardio

Cardio of choice: thirty minutes

Once again, this workout plan was created for my specific body type, frame and needs. It was tailored specifically for me and proved to show results. This plan may not work for everyone due to the complexities or uniqueness of every body type and needs. Be sure to check with your doctor before starting an exercise program.

Each week presented a unique challenge and continually tested my strength and willpower. Willpower can be extraordinary when faced with adversity and the desire to be well. For eight weeks, I worked tirelessly to "burn off sugar" in my body. To keep myself motivated I often had to refer to the saying, where there is a will, there is a way. I also placed a reminder on the wall of my home gym that reads, "Strength is a lack of Weakness" and "Weakness is a lack of Strength." Of course, I strived to embrace the first every single day.

When I started this process, Dolly performed a body composition measurement that revealed an estimated body fat at of 31.9 percent; ninety days later, my body fat had plummeted to 18.2 percent, resulting in a fourteen-pound weight loss and gaining five pounds of muscle.

20

Conclusion

ACCORDING TO MAINSTREAM medical science, once you have been diagnosed with diabetes you will always have it. If you return to your old eating habits and routines the diabetes will re-appear. They refer to miracles as a "hypothesis," as you will read in a letter to the editor in the appendix. We see this time and time again: mainstream medical science exclaim that researchers have either made a mistake or have no explanation for a given phenomenon, instead of acknowledging there is a God who heals. According to religious beliefs, God can heal diseases; for people of faith, there is something that God requires of all who ask for miracles to be manifested in their lives no matter what it is they are praying for. That requirement is simple "you must believe." Jesus did not perform many miracles in his own town because of the unbelief of those who knew him back home (Matthew 13:53–58).

Finally, the day had come to go get the results of my ninety-day follow-up blood test. November 30 2018, was that day, and I was ready. The night before had been a night of hope, high expectations, and anxiousness. After all, I did the work, I prayed day and night, and I followed both my nutritionist's and personal trainer's instructions. I remember thinking to myself that this journey had been a tough fight and I had done all I could do. I remembered how my daily blood sugar test would fluctuate and how much it had frustrated me in the beginning. Then I remembered who was in control and that this was for God's glory. I knew that everything was going to be okay, because the battle was not mine; it was the Lord's.

I was sitting in the doctor's office, waiting that November 30th morning. I knew that he and his staff were aware I never took the diabetes medication he'd prescribed to get my blood sugar under control. My thoughts were racing just thinking about the results, I couldn't contain my thoughts.

My doctor finally walked into the room and for some reason, the topic of my results seemed to take longer than usual. He sat down, began to talk about the weather and random things. This went on for what seemed to me as an eternity. I began to wonder if he'd forgotten what I was there for. He was smiling and talking and talking and smiling. I was literally losing my mind at this point. I desperately wanted to hear my blood test results. All of a sudden, he smiled and said, "I don't know what you did, but whatever you did worked." He began to read my results, one by one. He said, "Everything is normal (triglycerides, kidney function, vitamin D, cholesterol), and you are not diabetic anymore; what did you do? How did you accomplish this? Tell me; I need to know. In all of my years of practice, I have never witnessed such success. Can you write down everything you did so I can use it for my patients?"

"Wow!" I said. I was beyond thrilled, smiling ear to ear, I couldn't contain my excitement. I was jumping for joy inside. I answered his question by pointing up and with tears of joy in my eyes, I said to him, "It was God who healed me. It was the Lord."

He smiled, hugged me and restated, "Please write everything

down and share it with me." As I left his office, I immediately called my wife and mom. They were each so thrilled to hear such great news, relieved that this disease no longer lived in my body, controlled my life and proud of my triumph.

I then called my pastor, Bruce Klepp and talked about this miracle for more than twenty-five minutes. You see, earlier that morning, (prior to receiving the test results) I attended a meeting with Pastor Klepp, and I told him after the meeting that I was on my way to get my test results after three months of being diagnosed with diabetes. I explained to him about how Pastor Ed had prayed for me when he came down from Alaska. Pastor Klepp didn't know what I was struggling with until after that meeting that morning. He immediately laid hands on me and asked the Lord for a favorable blessing and a good report.

On the morning of November 30, 2018, my 90-day follow-up visit revealed a normal blood sugar level and a Hemoglobin A1c of 5 percent. Remember what I said at the beginning of my story, a normal Hemoglobin A1c is 5.7 percent or under. TO GOD BE THE GLORY! Hallelujah and Amen.

21

A Prayer Poem of Thanks for Healing

written by the author

My redeemer lives, and this I know.
The word of God tells me so.
He waits for us each day to worship him and pray.
He hears our prayers, as promised in his
word. Pray with all your heart,
and your prayer will be heard. I have lived
God's goodness and healing touch.
I have been healed, and I thank him so very
much. It's hard sometimes to pray
and believe, but he promises: whatever
we ask for, we will receive.
In his name, we pray to receive. In his
name, we pray and must believe.

Faith is not doubt and disbelief, which
robs your blessing like a thief.
Oh Lord my God, Father and Son, in heaven
and on earth, let your will be done.
Let your spirit come, Lord, and dwell in
me. Open mine eyes that I may see
that the Lord my God has set me free from
pain, sickness, and infirmity.
Thank you, Lord my God, for healing me.
Thank you, Lord my God, for this victory.
My arms and hands I will raise to give you
all the glory, honor, and praise.
Help me, Lord, to follow your ways
that I may be blessed [pause]
for the rest of my earthly days. Amen.

I give all the glory to the Lord my God. I declare victory
in the name of Jesus. Lord God, Jehovah Joshua Messiah,
I give you praise and glorify your name. Amen.

I encourage everyone: no matter the situation, no matter the
struggle, my story proves that God is a healer. If you have
faith and do your part to put the work in, you can and will
come out victorious and glorify his name in all you do.

For I know the plans I have for you, plans to
prosper you and not to harm you, plans to give
you hope and a future. (Jeremiah 29:11 NKJV)

Appendix

THE FOLLOWING IS a personal inquiry and editorial response from a well-known magazine known for its health publications. I tried to bring my story to the world via their magazine, however they were not interested in sharing my truth.

A Letter to an Editor

Dear editor,

My name is Herb McArthur. I am writing my story about how I overcame type 2 diabetes in ninety days. On August 31, 2018, I was diagnosed with an A1c of 8.8 and a blood sugar level of 246. I refused to take the diabetes medication, because I'd read that it could cause pancreatic cancer. What I did over the next ninety days without medication resulted in a normal blood sugar level and an A1c of 5.0 or 5 percent, as indicated in blood work taken on November 30, 2018. All documented and verified in my medical test results. My doctor called it a miracle, my pastors said the same. I want the world to know how this was accomplished because I want people to know that they can reverse this disease. How can you help me get this story out? How can you help me make a difference?

Sincerely,
Herbert McArthur

The Editor's Response

Dear Mr. McArthur:
Thanks for your email! And wonderful news about your diabetes.

Our publications adhere to mainstream medical wisdom, so technically, we don't ascribe to the hypothesis that diabetes can be *cured or reversed*. We do believe, however, that it can be well managed.

That said, if you have lifestyle tips you'd like to share we may be able to include them in upcoming diabetes guides.

Thanks again!
████████████

Editor in Chief
Health Monitor

People with type 2 diabetes who are able to get their HbA1c below 42 mmol/mol (6%) without taking diabetes medication are said to have reversed or resolved their diabetes.

—www.diabetes.co.uk https://www.diabetes.
co.uk/reversing-diabetes.html

Exercise Illustrations

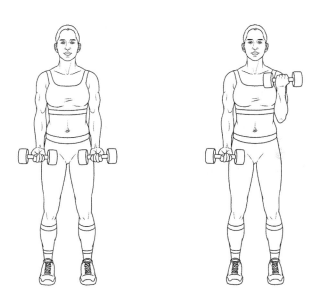

Alternating dumbbell curls

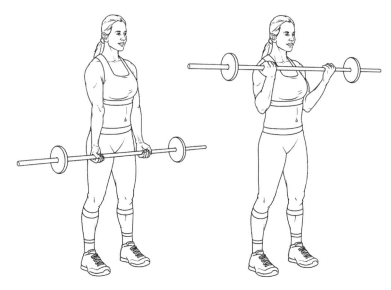

Barbell curls biceps

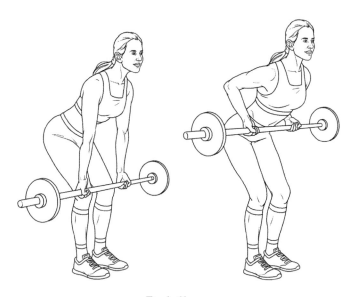

Barbell rows

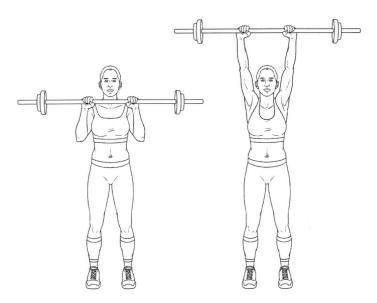

Barbell shoulder press

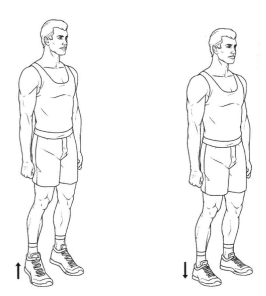

Calf-raises-exercise

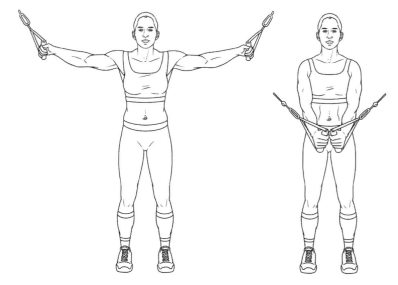

Chest cable cross

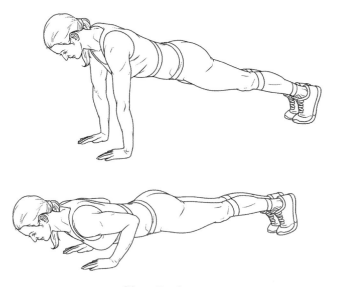

Chest Push ups

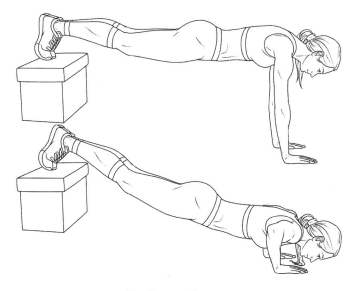

Decline push ups

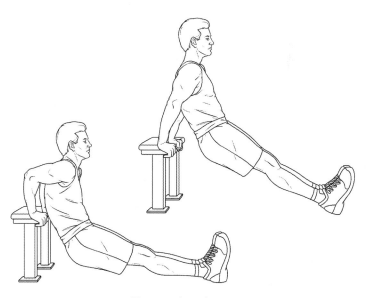

Dips on bench

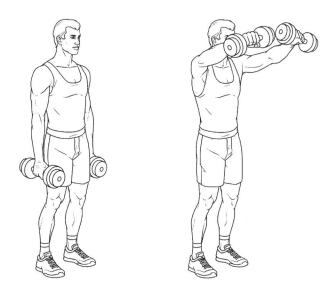

Dumbbell frontal raises

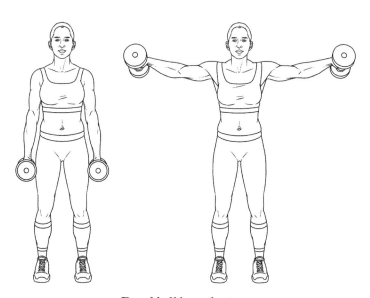

Dumbbell lateral raises

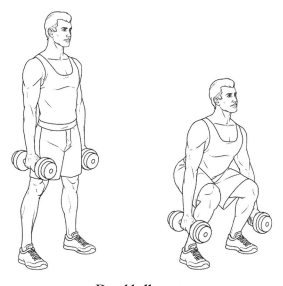

Dumbbell squats

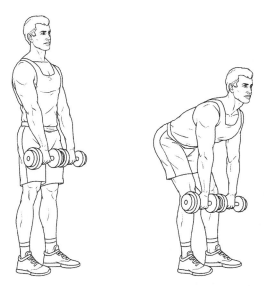

Dumbbell_Stiff_Leg_Deadlifts

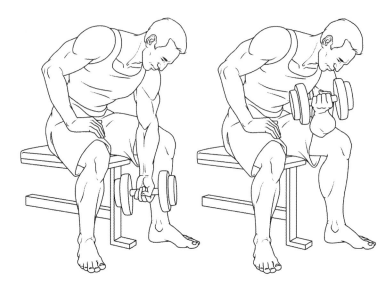

Dumbbell-Concentration-Curl

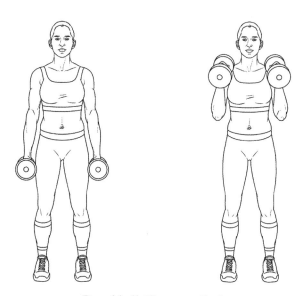

Dumbbell-Hammer-Curls

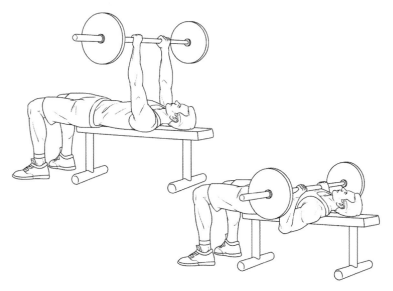

Flat barbell bench press

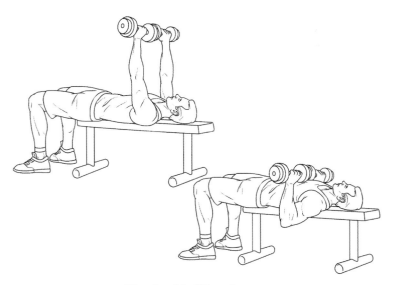

Flat dumbbell bench press

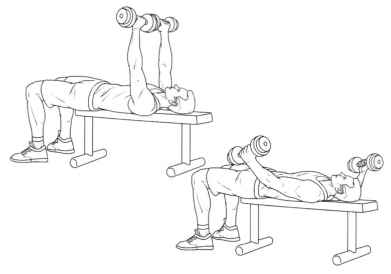

Flat dumbbell fly

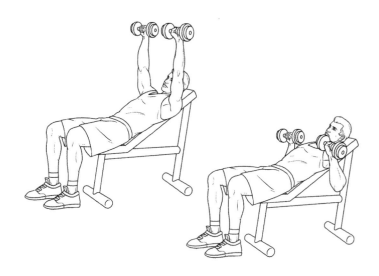

Incline dumbbell bench press

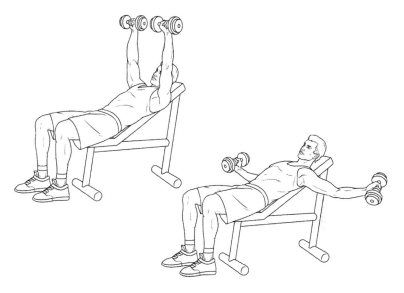

Incline dumbbell chest fly

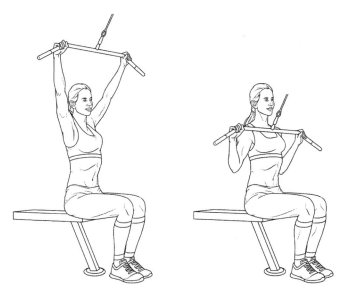

lat-pull-down

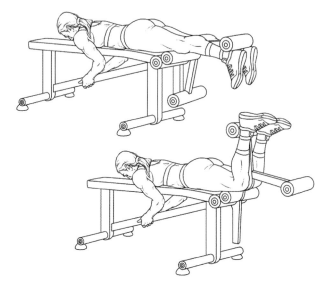

Leg-curl

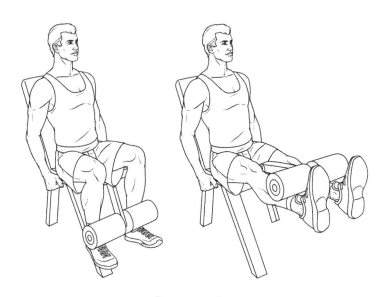

Leg-extension

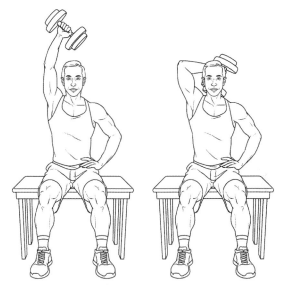

One arm triceps dumbbell overhead

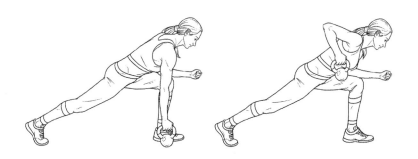

One-arm-row

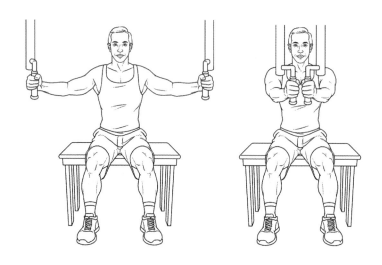

Pectoral fly

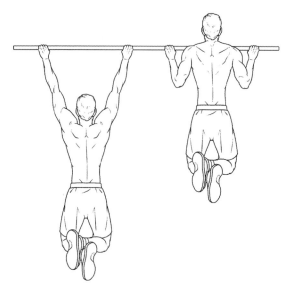

Pull ups

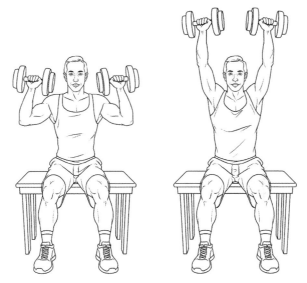

Seated dumbbell shoulder press

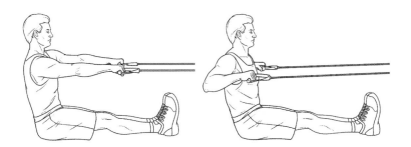

Seated rows

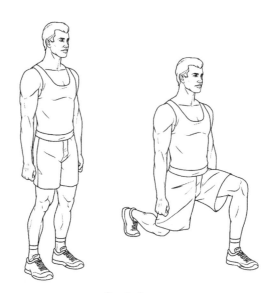

Static lunges

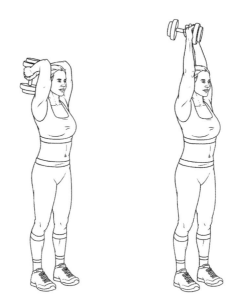

Triceps dumbbell overhead

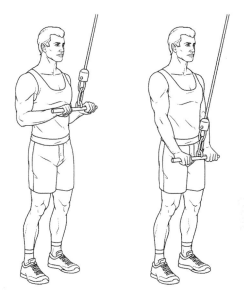

Triceps push down with bar

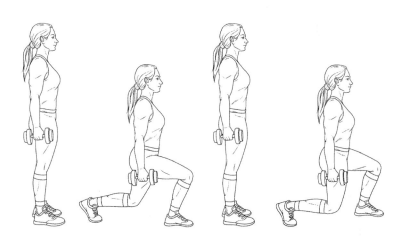

Walking lunges

References

"Bitter Melon and Diabetes." *Diabetes.co.uk*. The Global Diabetes Community. https://www.diabetes.co.uk/natural-therapies/bitter-melon.html.

Diabetes.co.uk: The Global Diabetes Community. www.diabetes.co.uk.

"Get Enough Sleep." *Everyday Healthy Eating*, July 18, 2019. https://healthfinder.gov/HealthTopics/Category/everyday-healthy-living/mental-health-and-relationship/get-enough-sleep.

Healthline. www.healthline.com.

Hopkins Medicine. www.hopkinsmedicine.org.

"How Stress Affects Blood Sugar Levels," 2019. https://glucerna.com/why-glucerna/how-stress-affects-blood-sugar-levels.

Martino, E. World Health Organization. 2016.

Mayo Clinic. www.mayoclinic.org.

Parsley, Rod (@RealRodParsley). Various posts. Twitter, 2015.

School of Public Health. Harvard University. hsph.harvard.edu.

Spritzer, Franziska. "The 16 Best Foods to Control Diabetes." *Healthline*, June 3, 2017. https://www.healthline.com/nutrition/16-best-foods-for-diabetics.

Tufts Medicare Preferred. www.tuftsmedicarepreferred.org.

Printed in the United States
By Bookmasters